MEDICOLEGAL DEATH INVESTIGATION FIELD GUIDE

**Investigation Unit
Cuyahoga County Medical Examiner's Office**

ISBN: 978-1-54390-651-6 (print)
ISBN: 978-1-54390-652-3 (ebook)

CONTENTS

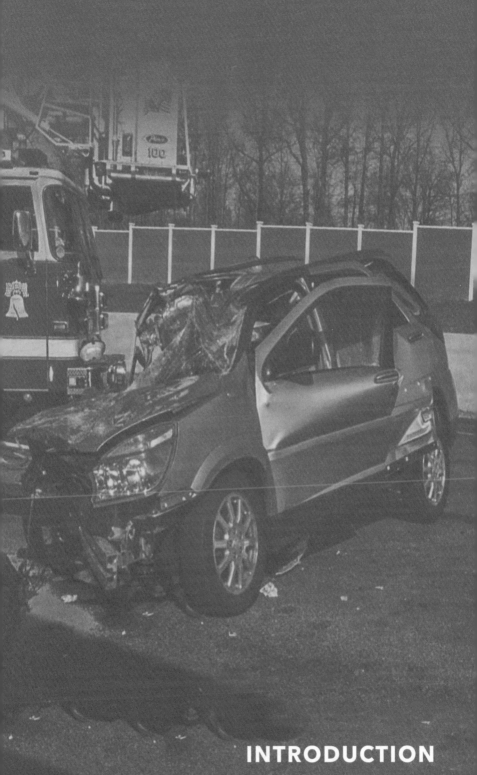

INTRODUCTION

INTRODUCTION

This guide is primarily meant for field use; however, much of the content is applicable to the investigation of deaths in which there is no scene visit. The guide is divided into three sections. Section I, the *Initial Notification*, consists of basic information to be obtained on all cases and a series of questions regarding the circumstances, death scene, body, and history (decedent profile) which are used to establish jurisdiction and serves as the foundation of every investigation. Information in the *Initial Notification* may be obtained during the initial phone call and at the death scene. Section II includes a list of *General Medicolegal Death Scene Investigative Procedures* to be performed in the majority of cases and a list of *Scene Safety Considerations*. Section III, *Scene Types*, covers *Indicators,* specific *Key Questions*, *Scene Procedures,* and *Red Flags* for a number of different case types. One death may have a number of *Applicable Scene Types* which are supplements to the information obtained in the *Initial Notification*.

A series of *Indicators* are presented for the majority of Scene Types. Indicators are signs (physical findings) or reasons (circumstances or history) to suspect a particular case type. Indicators are developed during the initial notification and scene investigation.

A list of *Key Questions* for each case type are intended to elicit positive or negative answers to pertinent aspects of the cause, manner and circumstances of death. Not all questions will be applicable in every case. Whenever possible, investigators should assert the negative, for example, "no alcohol or illicit drugs were found". What is absent from the scene is often as important as what is present.

A checklist of *Scene Procedures* are specific actions to be performed for each type of case to ensure a complete investigation.

Red Flags (⚑) are signs that an alternative cause or manner of death should be considered.

Applicable Scene Types are associated scene types that may be triggered by red flags, shared indicators, or comparable circumstances.

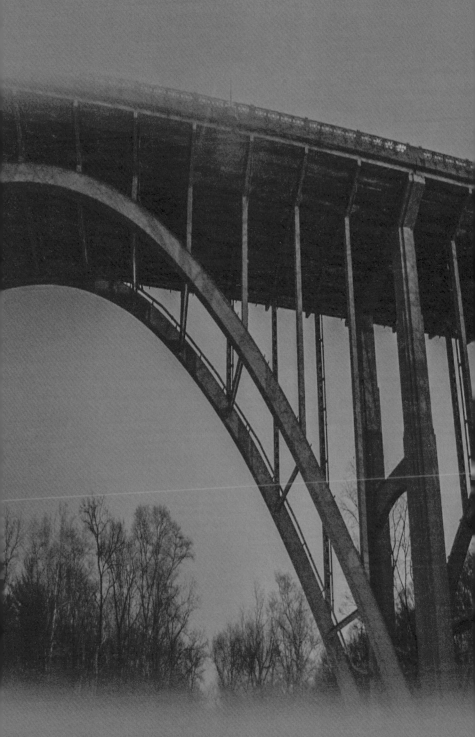

SECTION I

SECTION I
INITIAL NOTIFICATION

Reporting and Responding Agency Information

1. Date and time of notification
2. Agency and district
   a. Reportee Name, Rank and Badge number
      i. Phone number in the field
   b. Report or Incident number
3. Record same from other responding agencies
4. Emergency Medical Services
   a. Agency, unit number
   b. Time of call and time of death
   c. Pronouncing physician

Decedent Demographics

1. Full legal name
2. Date of birth
3. Race and sex
4. Marital status
5. Social security number
6. Home address

Identification

1. Has the decedent been positively identified?

    a.   Tentative identification may be appropriate in cases of decomposition, disfiguring facial trauma, thermal injuries, and multiple fatality incidents.

    b.   Jurisdiction is automatically accepted on all unidentified decedents.

2. By what means was positive identification made?

    a.   Record the name, relationship and contact information of the person making identification.

Legal Next of Kin (NoK)

1. Are there family members present?

    a.   Who is the legal NoK (see hierarchy below)?

        i.   Record name and relationship

        ii. Record phone number(s) and street address

    b.   Has the NoK been notified? When and by whom?

2. If NoK is unknown, what attempts have been made to locate family?

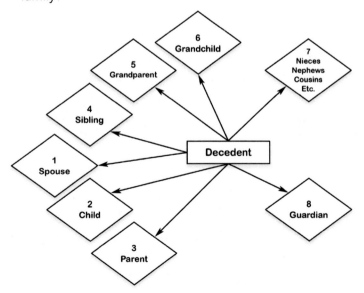

Circumstances (Pre and Post-Discovery)

1. When and where was the decedent last known alive, by whom, in-person or by phone?

    a. What was he/she doing at that time?

    b. Did the decedent have any complaints or symptoms? Specify.

2. Was the incident/death witnessed, by whom, and what happened?

3. Was the body found, by whom, and why were they looking for the decedent?

4. Does the decedent live alone? List occupants by relationship.

5. Has the **body** been moved, by whom, and why?

6. What manner of death does this appear to be and why?

Scene

1. Record the address and specify the place of death (work, home or other).

2. Is the body indoors or outdoors?

3. Was the residence secured?

    a. **Locked** means the interior of the residence is inaccessible without a key.

    b. **Secured** means access is restricted by an internal mechanism.

4. Are any of the following present; illicit drugs, paraphernalia or **excessive** alcohol?

5. Were any prescriptions found? Any near the body?

    a. Record names of prescriptions and prescribing physicians.

      b. Are any of the prescriptions narcotics or psychiatric medications?

          i.   Record the date filled and count (are they appropriate?)

      c. Are prescription quantities consistent with dosage prescribed?

6.   Is there evidence to suggest the decedent's activities prior to death? Describe.

7.   Are there signs of foul play?

      a. Unexplained forced entry, overturned furniture, ransacking, or missing personal property.

8.   How has the **scene** been altered, by whom, and why?

      a. Example: Police removed firearm from decedent's hand.

9.   Are there environmental concerns?

      a. What is the temperature?

      b. Are utilities functioning?

      c. Any fumes or potential sources of CO?

      d. Is the scene safe to enter?

          i.   If no, why?

Body

1.   What was the original location and position of the body?

      a. Does it appear the decedent fell or collapsed?

      b. Is the body pinned, wedged, or restrained?

2.   Any obvious trauma or blood loss? Describe.

3.   Any signs of decomposition? Describe.

Medical History

1.   What is the medical history and how was it obtained?

    a.   Does the history include:

        i.   Recent or remote injuries?

           1.   If yes – when, where and how did injuries occur?

               a.   Where was the decedent treated?

               b.   Any complications or lingering effects?

        ii.   Recent hospitalizations, surgeries or dental work? Explain.

        iii. Substance abuse or rehab? Specify.

        iv. Mental health conditions?

           1.   Suicide attempts / ideations?

2.   Obtain the name and contact information for all treating physicians.

    a.   Who is the primary care physician (PCP)?

    b.   Have any of the physicians been contacted?

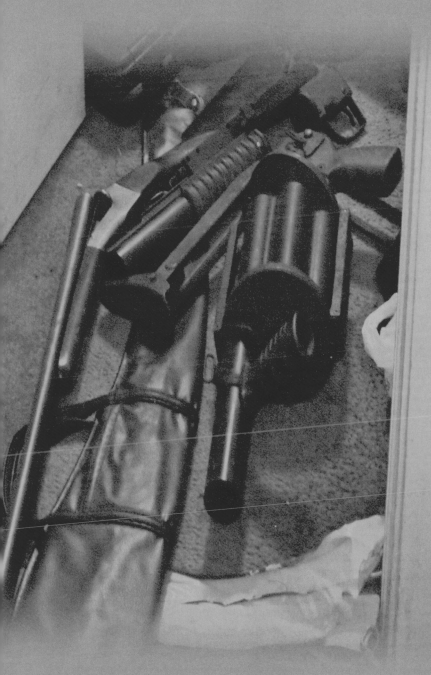

SECTION II

SECTION II
GENERAL MEDICOLEGAL
DEATH SCENE INVESTIGATIVE
PROCEDURES

CCMEO endorses the recommended practices and procedures contained in the National Institute of Justice's publication, *"Death Investigation: A Guide for the Scene Investigator: Technical Update" (2011)*.

The following practices and procedures are required in every death scene investigation.

Scene

1.   Obtain 8 minimum photographs.

    a.   Whiteboard

       i.   Single image of the dry erase board containing the date, decedent's name, scene address, and investigator's initials.

    b.   Exterior

       i.   An overall photograph of the home, building, roadway, or other location where the decedent is located.

    c.   Address

       i.   House or building number, a sign containing the name or address of the building/complex, or street signs indicating the nearest intersection or serving as a landmark. When documenting a death scene at an apartment building or hotel, a separate photograph should be taken of the unit door.

d. Overalls (2)

    i. Full-length views of the decedent from opposing vantage points. An overall may also be of a motor vehicle if the body was not ejected or has not been removed.

e. Mugshot

    i. A portrait photo of only the decedent's face. Consider at least one image where any disfiguring injuries are minimized in the event the photo is needed for visual identification.

f. Removal

    i. Single photo of the floor, ground, or other surface immediately below the decedent upon his/her removal.

g. Tag

    i. Single photo showing the serialized tag sealing the two body bag zippers.

2. Record the scene temperature.

3. Note the presence or absence of illicit drugs and/or paraphernalia.

a. Collect drugs and paraphernalia in non-homicide cases (unless otherwise directed).

4. Note the presence or absence of prescription medications.

a. Collect prescription medications in non-homicide cases.

5. Note the presence of excessive alcohol, or absence of alcohol.

6. Note the presence or absence of foul play.

7. Document medical records, bills, devices and equipment.

   a. Record the most recent readings on glucose and/or blood pressure monitors.

   b. Note medical, dental and insurance provider information (as necessary).

8. Document items that assist in narrowing the postmortem interval.

   a. Newspapers, mail, phone, receipts, etc.

9. Note the presence of bloodstains in relationship to the body.

10. Search for items useful in identifying / notifying NoK and establishing indigence.

   a. Collect financial, insurance, military documents, and/or last will.

11. Search for and collect driver's license or photo identification if not on the body.

12. Lock and seal the residence and collect the key.

   a. Residence should be sealed when;

      i. decedent lives alone,

      ii. suspected homicide,

      iii. suspected carbon monoxide or hazardous environment,

      iv. family has yet to be notified.

13. Ask police to perform a criminal history check and note results.

14. Provide information pamphlet to family.

Body

1. Describe clothing including any defects.
2. Photograph all personal effects.
3. Assess and describe rigor, livor, and body temperature.
4. Describe decomposition changes.
5. Describe injuries in a conservative manner.
6. Note and photograph bloodstains.

SECTION II
SCENE SAFETY
CONSIDERATIONS

Medicolegal Death Investigators (MDI) must operate with heightened awareness of potential hazards at death scenes. The most common hazards are safety, biological, physical, and chemical. When a Safety Officer has been designated (Fire, Explosion, HAZMAT or Disaster), obtain instructions for the appropriate level of Personal Protective Equipment (PPE) and obtain clearance to enter the scene. For a normal scene investigation, minimize risk of injury at the scene by adhering to the following practices;

1. Always address safety and security concerns with first responders before entering.

2. Never hesitate to request animal control, fire department or HAZMAT.

3. Use Universal Precautions.

4. Wear appropriate Personal Protective Equipment (PPE) including footwear.

5. Put on (don) shoe covers when bodily fluids are present on the floor.

6. Use double-gloves and change the outer gloves when soiled.

7. Remove (doff) PPE slowly and deliberately in the correct sequence.

    a. Outer gloves, goggles/face shield, gown, shoe covers, mask or respirator, inner gloves.

    b. Shoe covers must be removed with gloved hands.

8. Use a flashlight or arrange for proper lighting.

9. Wear a high-visibility reflective vest when investigating traffic fatalities.

10. Know your agency's Exposure Control Plan.

11. Use appropriate containers when collecting items.

12. Allow patrol officers to clear and secure firearms before examination/handling.

13. Do not contaminate re-usable or jointly used equipment and tools including county vehicles. Always clean the equipment and tools after each use.

14. Follow your agency's written safety procedures.

Placed

Found

SECTION III

SECTION III
SCENE TYPES

HOMICIDE

<u>Indicators</u>

There are a number of physical and circumstantial indicators of a potential Homicide. Any time Homicide is suspected, the following questions should be asked.

<u>Key Questions</u>

1. Are there signs of struggle / physical altercation? Explain.
2. Are there defense wounds?
3. Does it appear the body has been moved / dumped?
4. Is there evidence that attempts were made to conceal the homicide?
5. If not otherwise addressed, what specifically makes the death suspicious?

<u>Scene Procedures</u>

1. Perform minimal handling of the body and clothing.
2. Roll the body onto a clean white sheet prior to a superficial examination.
3. Leave wrappings and bindings in place.
4. Photograph each hand (palmar and dorsal surfaces) without manipulating the fingers.

5. Secure the hands in clean paper bags with rubber bands or tape.

6. Never remove clothing at the scene.

7. Place the shrouded body directly into the body bag.

8. Evidence in a homicide investigation that's not on the body must be collected by the police.

9. Refer to specific Scene Types for additional procedures.

Applicable Scene Types

◆ Homicide could be a possibility in many of the following Scene Types.

NATURAL

Indicators

The Medical Examiner accepts jurisdiction on Natural deaths when there is no known medical history; no attending physician; when the death initially presents as violent or suspicious; and when the body is decomposed. Scene findings may include prescriptions, over-the-counter medications, and supplements; medical records, devices, and equipment; and occasionally herbal remedies.

The primary investigative objective in an apparent Natural death is to include or exclude trauma (acute and remote), intoxication, and environmental injury as potential causes of death.

Key Questions

1. Complete the questions from the *Initial Notification*.

Scene Procedures

1. Follow General Medicolegal Death Scene Investigative Procedures.

🚩 Red-Flags

Body position (possible asphyxia); presence of visible trauma; alcohol, illicit drugs, or paraphernalia, commonly abused prescription drugs; discrepancies after prescription inventory; temperature extremes; exhaust fumes; APS or CPS history; multiple decubitus ulcers; neglect of care.

Applicable Scene Types

◆ Natural death should be considered as an Applicable Scene Type in most cases when there's no obvious trauma, source of intoxication, or fatal environments.

SUICIDE

Indicators

There are numerous physical, circumstantial, and historical indicators of Suicide. Anytime Suicide is suspected, the following questions should be asked.

Key Questions

1. Diagnosed mental health conditions?

2. Any medications for mental health conditions?

3. Ever hospitalized for mental health conditions? When, where, and why?

4. Previous suicide attempts? Describe.

   a. If treated, where?

5. Voiced explicit suicidal threats or ideations? Describe.

6. Significant life events, changes or losses?

    a. Employment, financial, relationship, legal problems, bullying. Specify.

7. Any recent (terminal) medical diagnoses?

8. Is the date of death of any significance? Specify.

9. Is there evidence suggesting arrangement of final affairs or giving away possessions?

    a. Ex: Organization of possessions and/or important documents.

10. Was a suicide note found? Including text or computer messages.

11. Is there a history of substance abuse?

Scene Procedures

1. Leave bindings in place.

2. Photograph suicide notes, text messages, and/or computer searches.

3. Collect suicide notes in accordance with agency protocols.

4. Photograph physical items that suggest arrangement of final affairs.

5. Photograph each hand (palmar and dorsal surfaces) without manipulating the fingers.

6. Secure the hands in clean paper bags with rubber bands or tape in all gunshot cases and suspicious hangings.

7. Refer to specific Scene Types for additional procedures.

Applicable Scene Types

◆ Suicide could be a possibility in many of the following Scene Types.

ABUSE OR NEGLECT OF AN ADULT

Homicide

Indicators

Physically or mentally disabled persons who depend on care from others are at risk for abuse or neglect. Be suspicious when there's a history of involvement with Adult Protective Services (APS). Indications of physical abuse include: use of restraints; unexplained or untreated injuries; and multiple injuries of different ages. Common indications of neglect include: malnutrition or dehydration; physically unclean or unkempt appearance; inadequate wound or medical care; inappropriate medication administration; and lack of food, water, utilities or basic safety precautions. Unexplained vaginal or anal bleeding are signs of possible sexual abuse.

Key Questions

1. To what extent was the decedent capable of self-care?

    a. Performs activities of daily living independently, requires some assistance, or requires total assistance.

    b. Ambulatory status / use of mobility aids?

2. Who is the primary caregiver and what is their relationship to the decedent?

    a. What is the caregiver's normal schedule or routine of care (i.e. 3 days per week)?

    b. When was the last home visit (date/time)?

    c. Is the home health aide certified?

        i. Self-employed or employed by an agency? What agency?

3. How and by whom are prescriptions administered?

4. Is adequate food and water available?

5. What is the caregiver's explanation for any observed signs of abuse or neglect?

6. Any allegation(s) of abuse or neglect made to APS in the past?

   a. Outcome of the investigation?

7. Any prior encounters with law enforcement at the home or with the involved parties?

8. Was the decedent sexually active?

Scene Procedures

1. Request detectives respond to the scene and perform a joint interview with caregiver(s).

2. Assess medications for compliance.

3. Photograph the condition of any medical dressings.

4. Photograph soiled clothing and/or bedding inconsistent with circumstances.

5. Photograph safety/medical equipment.

6. Photograph specific unsafe living conditions.

7. Photograph food supply (refrigerator, pantry).

Applicable Scene Types

◆ *Blunt Force Injuries*
◆ *Environmental Injuries*
◆ *Intoxication / Overdose*

ABUSE OR NEGLECT OF A CHILD OR ADOLESCENT

Homicide

Indicators

Children requiring continuous medical care are also at ele-vated risk for abuse or neglect by their primary caregiver. Developmentally disabled persons and wards of the State are reportable conditions and should be examined for signs of abuse or neglect. Be suspicious when there's a known history of involvement with Child Protective Services (CPS) and when signs of substance abuse are found at the residence. Indications of physical abuse include: use of restraints; unexplained or untreated injuries; and multiple injuries of different ages. Common indications of neglect include: malnutrition or dehy-dration; physically unclean or unkempt appearance; inadequate wound or medical care; inappropriate medication administra-tion; and lack of food, water, utilities or basic safety precautions. Unexplained vaginal or anal bleeding are signs of possible sexual abuse. Consider abuse or neglect when parents have a non-religious objection to autopsy in an otherwise unexpected death, or when siblings have died unexpectedly.

Key Questions

1. Who was in charge of caring for the decedent when found unresponsive or at the time of death?

    a. What is their relationship to the decedent?

2. Is the location a licensed daycare or other child care environ-ment? Name.

3. Was the decedent sick or behaving differently in the hours or days preceding death?

    a. If yes, ask for a detailed description.

4. Was the decedent unattended for any amount of time? Specify.

5. How many persons occupy the residence (specify the number of adults and children)?

6. How and by whom are prescriptions administered?

7. Is adequate food and water available?

8. What is the caregiver's explanation for any observed signs of abuse or neglect?

9. Any allegation(s) of abuse or neglect made to APS in the past?

    a. Outcome of the investigation?

10. Any prior encounters with law enforcement at the home or with the involved parties?

Scene Procedures

1. Request detectives respond to the scene and perform a joint interview with caregiver(s).

2. Assess medications (decedent and caregivers).

3. Photograph the condition of any medical dressings.

4. Photograph soiled clothing and/or bedding.

5. Photograph safety or medical equipment.

6. Photograph specific unsafe living conditions.

7. Photograph food supply (refrigerator, pantry).

Applicable Scene Types

♦ *Asphyxia*
♦ *Blunt Force Injuries*

- *Environmental Injuries*
- *Intoxication / Overdose*
- *Sudden Unexpected Infant Death Investigations (SUIDI)*

ASPHYXIA

CHEMICAL

Suicide, Accident, Homicide

Indicators

Chemical asphyxiants most likely encountered by MDI's in non-industrial deaths include Carbon Monoxide (CO) and Hydrogen Sulfide (H_2S). Be suspicious of H_2S when a decedent is found inside an enclosed vehicle parked in an isolated area. Hand-written or printed warning signs regarding poisonous gases may be affixed to the vehicle's windows. Household cleaning products and mixing containers may be present in the vehicle and the decedent may have blue-green lividity in an H_2S case. CO is discussed in the next section.

Key Questions

1. What type of toxic gas is suspected?
2. What chemicals were used to create the gas?
3. Did FD/HAZMAT obtain an initial reading of the environment?
   a. What were the results?
4. Was the body removed and/or decontaminated prior to ME arrival?

Scene Procedures

1. Do not approach the scene until the source has been identified and mitigated.

2. Request HAZMAT to extricate and decontaminate the body and clothing.

3. Photograph any posted or visible warning signs.

4. Photograph chemicals and containers.

5. Document attempts to seal the vehicle, such as taping the doors, windows, and/or air vents.

6. Request a HAZMAT incident report.

🚩 Red-Flags

Carbon monoxide; helium (He) or nitrogen (N); plastic bag over head.

Applicable Scene Types

◆ *Carbon Monoxide (CO)*
◆ *Asphyxia - Plastic Bag ("Final Exit")*
◆ *Suicide*

CARBON MONOXIDE (CO)

Suicide, Accident, Homicide

Indicators

Carbon monoxide poisoning produces lividity which is cherry-red in color. Death scenes may have multiple decedents including pets. Other occupants may be sickened and transported to a hospital. Be suspicious of CO poisoning in fall and winter when home heating is turned on for the first time and when gas-powered generators are used improperly.

Key Questions

1. What is the suspected source of the CO?

   a. Is there evidence of malfunctioning appliances or heating sources (Accident)?

   b. Is there an apparatus to divert the fumes (Suicide, Homicide)?

2. What was the CO level measured by fire department?

3. Was the scene ventilated? How?

4. Did the decedent(s) or other occupants have symptoms of exposure such as headaches, dizziness, nausea or vomiting?

5. Is there a CO detector in the home? Working?

Scene Procedures

1. Request local fire department measure the CO level and deem the scene safe to enter.

2. Photograph the source including any ventilation.

3. Lock and seal the property.

   a. Notify family that the fire department must provide clearance to enter the residence.

🚩 Red-Flags

The home has no gas utilities. Frozen bodies may also have cherry-red lividity. The CO level measured by the fire department is not considered toxic.

Applicable Scene Types

◆   *Suicide*

CARBON MONOXIDE (CO) - BODY INSIDE VEHICLE OR ENCLOSED SPACE

Suicide, Accident (rare)

Indicators

Medicolegal investigators should suspect CO whenever a body is discovered inside an enclosed space, like a garage, with vehicles or other gas-powered equipment present. In suicides, hoses or other apparatus may be attached to the tailpipe directing exhaust to the inside of the vehicle.

Key Questions

1.   Are keys in the ignition? What position?

  a.   If not, did someone remove the keys?

2.   Was a CO level obtained by the fire department? Results?

  a.   If not, was there an odor of exhaust upon discovery of the body?

3.   Was the scene ventilated prior to ME arrival? How?

Scene Procedures

1.   Request local fire department to measure CO level and deem the scene safe to enter.

2.   Touch the vehicle's hood or other gas-powered equipment to check relative temperature.

3.   Check and photograph the fuel gauge level without starting the vehicle.

4.   Photograph any mechanism used to divert exhaust fumes from tailpipe to the interior of the vehicle

5.   Photograph items used to seal exhaust fumes within the garage/enclosed space.

6.   Note where dead animals were taken (as applicable).

🚩 Red-Flags

No source of combustion.

Applicable Scene Types

◆   *Suicide*

COMPRESSION (TRAUMATIC)

Accident, Homicide

Indicators

With traumatic compression, normal respiration is impeded by a heavy object compressing the chest and/or abdomen. The decedent may also be buried (sand, grain bin, trench collapse). Physical signs of compression include congestion/cyanosis of the face, neck and upper chest, as well as petechiae and Tardieu spots.

Key Questions

1.   Was the incident witnessed? By whom? What happened?

2.   Was a heavy object compressing the neck, chest or abdomen?

3.   What was the known or estimated weight of the object?

4.   How was extrication made?

5. Was the decedent believed to be intoxicated? By what substance?

Scene Procedures

1. Photograph the object from eye-level and ground-level.

2. Photograph any signs or labels that provide details about the object.

3. Photograph any pattern injuries.

4. If the item has not been moved, measure the distance from the ground to the object to record the amount of space the body was compressed.

Applicable Scene Types

◆ *Motor Vehicle Accidents*
◆ *In-Custody - Restraints*
◆ *Sudden Unexpected Infant Death Investigations (SUIDI)*
◆ *Work-Related*

CHOKING

Accident, Homicide

Indicators

Choking should be part of the investigative differential diagnosis if the decedent collapsed/arrested while eating. In an unwitnessed death, investigators should consider the possibility of choking when food is discovered near the body.

Key Questions

1. What was the decedent eating?

2. Was the incident witnessed? By whom?

a. Did the decedent demonstrate signs of distress, or universal sign of choking (neck clutch)?

3. Does the decedent have MRDD, dementia, dysphagia or other neurological or physical disorder?

4. Was the decedent intoxicated?

5. Do they wear dentures or have poor dentition?

6. CHILDREN: Was the child playing while eating?

7. Did EMS suction/dislodge anything from the airway?

a. What was removed?

Scene Procedures

1. Do not remove material from the mouth.

2. Do not remove gag or tape over mouth (Homicide).

3. Photograph food on or near the body.

4. Photograph any dislodged food or material.

Red-Flags

No food present. Decedent had a G-tube or was unable to feed him or herself.

Applicable Scene Types

◆ *Abuse or Neglect of an Adult*
◆ *Abuse or Neglect of a Child or Adolescent*

HANGING

Suicide, Accident

Indicators

Physical signs of a hanging may include petechiae, protruding tongue, ligature furrow, and Tardieu spots. There is a distinct lividity pattern. The body should be suspended (fully or partially) unless cut down by family or first responders.

Key Questions

1. Is the body suspended or not?
   a. Partially or fully suspended?
2. Ligature cut or untied?
   a. By whom? How?
   b. Neck ligature removed? By whom?
3. What is the ligature?
   a. Is there a receipt for the purchase of this ligature?
4. Are there specific findings on the body (see indicators)?
   a. Were the hands bound? In front or behind?
5. What is the point of suspension (object and means of attachment)?
   a. What is the distance from the point of suspension to the floor?
   b. What is the distance from the point of suspension to the knot/neck?
   c. Are there signs of wear to indicate previous attempts (or autoerotic activity)?
   d. Was a platform (step-off) used?

6. Is there evidence this could be an accident? (autoerotic, hanging game)

Scene Procedures

1. Document the ligature, knots, and point of suspension.
2. Obtain measurements (key question #5).
3. Leave ligature in place around the neck.
    a. Leave clothing in place if entangled within ligature.
4. Collect portions of cut ligatures.
5. Use caution when bringing body down.
    a. Preserve the knot whenever possible
6. Photograph point at which ligature is anchored, the suspension point on the neck, and any knots
7. Photograph any step-off
8. Photograph the decedent's hands

Red-Flags

Orientation of the ligature furrow (horizontal could be strangulation); inconsistent postmortem changes (Homicide), hanging-game, illustrations or how-to materials, state of dress, bondage, bindings, pornographic materials, protective padding, mirrors, camera, fail-safe.

Applicable Scene Types

- *Asphyxia - Strangulation*
- *Autoerotic*
- *In-Custody*
- *Suicide*

AUTOEROTIC

Accident

Indicators

Autoerotic asphyxia should be considered when the decedent is found suspended with any of the following present: pornographic material, sex toys, a fail-safe mechanism, and evidence of previous/repeated use of the anchor point.

Key Questions

1. Does the suspension point show signs of wear to indicate previous autoerotic activity?
2. Is there protective padding between the ligature and the neck?
3. Are there signs of bondage?
4. Is there pornographic material or sex-toys?
5. Are there mirrors or cameras?
6. Is there a fail-safe (escape) mechanism?

Scene Procedures

1. Follow procedures for Hangings.
2. Leave ligature, bindings, and other contraptions in place.
3. Photograph any pornography, sex-themed products, or any indications of prior activity

Applicable Scene Types

◆ *Suicide*

PLASTIC BAG OR "FINAL EXIT"

Suicide

Indicators

Items found at the scene that suggest a plastic bag ("Final Exit") type suicide include: a plastic bag on or about the head, tank containing inert gases (He, N), hoses, and pills. Also, be mindful of literature that describes ending your life.

Key Questions

1. Was the plastic bag moved or removed?
2. How was the plastic bag secured to the neck?
3. Are there any medications on scene (prescription or over- the-counter)?
4. Was the tank on or off when the body was found?
   a. Empty or still running?
5. Are there receipts for the purchase of the equipment?
   a. When were the items purchased?

Scene Procedures

1. Ask the *finder* to describe their actions upon discovering the body.
2. Photograph the apparatus (plastic bag, hose(s), connectors, and tank).
   a. Photograph the orientation of the plastic bag around the head/neck.
3. Photograph pertinent literature or internet search history.
4. Leave the plastic bag and tubing in place.

5.   Clothing should be left in place as removal may displace plastic bag/apparatus.

6.   Collect the tank – try to keep the apparatus intact (if possible).

Applicable Scene Types

◆   *Intoxication / Overdose*
◆   *Suicide*

POSITIONAL

Accident, Homicide

Indicators

Infants, elderly/senile, obese, alcoholic or intoxicated persons are susceptible to positional asphyxia. Also, deaths in police custody during restraint may be attributed to body position. The decedent could be wedged or pinned. Petechiae, Tardieu spots, and cyanosis may be observed.

Key Questions

1.   Is the body in a position that impedes the normal process of respiration? Describe.

2.   Has the body been moved from its original position?

3.   Was the decedent believed to be intoxicated?

4.   Does the decedent have a medical condition that could inhibit self-extrication?

Scene Procedures

1.   Photograph the position of the head, neck and chest from multiple angles including "ground-level".

2.   Photograph any objects/restraints on the decedent's mouth, nose, neck, or chest.

3.   Obtain measurements as applicable (wedged, trapped, or pinned).

Applicable Scene Types

◆   *In-Custody*
◆   *Motor Vehicle Accidents*
◆   *Sudden Unexpected Infant Death Investigations (SUIDI)*
◆   *Work-Related*

STRANGULATION

Homicide, Suicide (rare), Accident (children)

MANUAL

Indicators

If the decedent was conscious while being manually strangled, investigators should expect to see defensive injuries or signs of a violent struggle. Physical findings on the body may include: fingermarks (crescent-shaped marks) on the neck, chin or jaw; congestion/cyanosis of the face and neck; and facial and conjunctival petechiae.

LIGATURE

Indicators

If the decedent was conscious while being strangled with a ligature, investigators should expect to see defensive injuries or signs of a violent struggle. Physical findings on the body may include: a horizontal ligature furrow; congestion/cyanosis of the face and neck; and facial and conjunctival petechiae.

Key Questions

1. Is there a ligature mark or other injuries to the neck?

   a. How is the ligature mark oriented?

2. What was used or suspected to have been used to strangle the decedent?

3. Is a ligature present on the body or in the immediate area?

4. Is there a history of domestic violence?

5. Is there an active restraining / protection order?

Scene Procedures

1. Obtain a history of events from the lead detective.

2. If the death is not initially recognized as a potential strangulation and the MDI observes indicators, request detectives respond to the scene.

3. Examine the face and eyes for petechiae and note the presence or absence.

4. Photograph items on the neck including necklaces, scarves, etc.

5. Leave ligatures in place around the neck.

6. Follow agency protocols for swabbing the neck or ligature for suspect DNA.

   a. CCMEO Trace Evidence personnel perform this procedure at the office.

🚩 Red-Flags

Ligature furrow consistent with a hanging. In rare occasions, a decedent may tighten a large zip-tie around his or her own neck in a suicide. Children may participate in asphyxial games that could result in accidental death.

Applicable Scene Types

◆ *Hanging*
◆ *Suicide*

BLUNT FORCE INJURIES

Indicators

Blunt force injuries are caused by a number of different mechanisms including physical assaults, falls, jumping from heights, and motor vehicle accidents. Physical findings include abrasions, battle's sign, contusions, lacerations, and raccoon eyes. Blunt objects may leave patterns on the skin.

ASSAULT WITH A BLUNT OBJECT

Homicide

Key Questions

1. Was this a physical fight or was a blunt object used?

    a. What is it?

    b. Where was it found?

    c. Has it been moved since it was found? By whom? Why?

    d. Is there apparent blood on it?

2. Are there patterned injuries? Generally describe.

Scene Procedures

1. Photograph the suspected blunt object.

2. Obtain measurements of the object.

3. Photograph similar objects present at the scene (as applicable).

4. Never remove an object that is embedded in the body.

    a. Cover the handle/exposed end with a clean paper bag or envelope.

FALLS DOWN STAIRS

Accident, Homicide

Indicators

Whenever a body is found on the stairs or at the base of the staircase, investigators must suspect blunt force injuries.

Key Questions

1. Was the incident witnessed?

    a. Was anyone else home at the time?

2. Was the decedent intoxicated?

3. Does the decedent have a medical condition that affects mobility?

4. How many steps make up the staircase?

5. What type of surface is on the staircase (wood, carpet)? Specify.

6. Is there a handrail or rails?

    a. What is the condition of the handrail (normal, loose, damaged)?

7. Is there damage to the steps or walls? Describe.

8. Were there slip/trip hazards or items on the steps? Describe.

9. Was the decedent wearing footwear?

a. What type?

b. Tied or untied?

Scene Procedures

1. Photograph from top and bottom of stairs to capture overall condition of stairs, handrails, and walls.

2. Photograph objects or hazards on the stairs.

3. Obtain a close-up photo of any damage to steps, handrails or walls.

4. If there's a motorized chair lift, describe its condition.

⚑ Red-Flags

Injuries inconsistent with a simple fall; Injuries to multiple planes of the body and different sides of the head; Injuries to protected areas like the neck and inner thighs; Projected bloodstains higher on the walls or the ceiling than would be expected.

Applicable Scene Types

◆ *Assault with a Blunt Object*
◆ *Intoxication / Overdose*

FALLS FROM STANDING

Accident, Natural

Indicators

Determine whether the incident was a true fall or a collapse. Persons with certain medical conditions are subject to collapse (syncope).

Key Questions

1. History of falls?

2. Were any slip or trip hazards identified (animals, wet floor, ice, curb, etc.)?

3. Did the decedent strike his/her head? Lose consciousness?

4. Physical disabilities that may have contributed?

    a. Does the decedent use or need assistance ambulating (cane, walker, wheelchair)?

5. Was the decedent wearing footwear? What type? Tied or untied?

6. Did they have any symptoms or complaints before being found down?

7. Was the decedent drinking or intoxicated when they fell?

Scene Procedures

Follow General Medicolegal Death Scene Investigative Procedures to properly document this type of scene.

FALLS OR JUMP FROM HEIGHT

Accident, Suicide, Homicide

Indicators

The decedent is usually found at the base of a building, under a bridge or below a cliff.

Key Questions

1. Is this a suspected fall, jump or push?

2. From what height did the fall occur (point of departure)?

3. What is the landing surface?

4. Intermediary objects between the suspected point of departure and landing surface?

5. Were barriers or safeguards in place? Were safeguards normal or defective?

6. Were there slip/trip hazards?

7. Is there video footage?

8. What is the length and type of ladder (step or extension)?

9. Does the ladder appear normal, damaged or defective?

JUMPERS

Suicide

<u>Key Questions</u>

1. Is the decedent's vehicle parked nearby?

2. How did the decedent gain access to the point of departure?

3. Was a suicide note found on the body, in the vehicle, or inside the apartment (as applicable)?

<u>Scene Procedures</u>

1. Photograph barriers and safeguards including any damage.

2. Photograph from suspected point of departure down to landing surface (if safe to do so).

3. Photograph from landing surface up to suspected point of departure (i.e. rooftop, platform).

4. Photograph any intermediate items that the decedent may have struck while falling.

    a. Photograph clothing that may have come off during descent.

5. Photograph footwear.

6. Photograph personal safety equipment, connections or OSHA required equipment.

7. Photograph ladder damage, defects and warning labels.

8. Determine the distance between the land site and building line. (If applicable)

9. If suspicious, secure the hands in clean paper bags with rubber bands or tape.

🚩 Red-Flags

Ladder under/near power sources, electrical tools in use, work related (safety requirements)

Applicable Scene Types

◆   *Suicide*

DROWNING

Accident, Suicide, Homicide

Indicators

There must be a history of submersion including the nose and mouth. The body/face should be wet. A foam cone may be present. Human remains discovered in a body of water may have blunt force injuries caused by water current and impact with the ground at the bottom; and postmortem changes caused by aquatic insects and animals.

TUBS

Key Questions

1.   Who found the body?

2.   Was water in the tub?

3.   Was the water running?

4.   What was the position of the body?

   a.   Were the nose and mouth submerged?

5.   Did the "finder" remove the body?

6.   Did the "finder" drain the water?

7.   Are there other items or articles in the tub (clothing, towels, or shower curtain)?

Scene Procedures

1.   Ask the "finder" to demonstrate their actions upon finding the body.

2.   Describe the tub, status of the drain and the presence of any safety devices.

3.   Note electrical sources/devices near the tub.

4.   If water is present, describe the clarity, depth, and temperature.

   a.   If empty, note presence of a line of demarcation ("water line").

5.   If the body is still in the tub, photograph the face to demonstrate whether or not the nose and mouth are/were submerged.

🏴 Red-flags

Lividity inconsistent with body position; body removed from tub and not wet; area around body is not wet; history of major depression or suicide attempts; presence of illicit drugs, alcohol or commonly abused prescriptions

Applicable Scene Types

◆ *Intoxication / Overdose*
◆ *Seizures*
◆ *Suicide*

POOLS

Key Questions

1. Was the incident witnessed or was the body discovered?
2. How long was the decedent submerged?
3. What activities, if any, were they doing in the water?
4. Is the pool private or public?
5. Was a certified lifeguard on duty?
6. Is the water level appropriate?
7. What was the decedent's swimming ability?

Scene Procedures

1. Note any electrical sources/devices near the pool.
2. Describe the configuration of the pool (dimensions and depths).
3. Describe any equipment in and around pool (fencing, safety devices and signage, steps, ladders).
4. Describe the clarity, depth, and temperature of the water

🚩 Red-flags

Body is not wet; history of major depression or past suicide attempts; presence of illicit drugs, alcohol or commonly abused prescriptions

Applicable Scene Types

◆ Intoxication / Overdose
◆ Seizures
◆ Suicide

BODIES OF WATER

Key Questions

1. Was the incident witnessed or was the body discovered?
2. How long was the decedent submerged?
3. What activities, if any, were they doing in the water?
4. How was the decedent recovered from the water?
5. Was the decedent partially or fully submerged when found?
6. What is the type of bottom (if known)?
7. Were there warning signs posted?
8. What is the decedent's known swimming ability?
9. Was the decedent restrained in anyway?
10. Was there any trauma to the body?
11. Was there washer woman skin?
12. Is the clothing consistent with location/circumstances found?
    a. Is the clothing / body wet or dry?
13. If the decedent was swimming with others, did anyone else have difficulty?

Scene Procedures

1. Describe the water (clarity, color, depth, temperature, and current).
2. Describe the immediate area (slopes, points of entry).
3. Obtain an estimated depth of the water where the body was found.
4. Request photos and report from the agency that recovered the body.
5. Photograph the point of entry (if known).

🏳 Red-Flags

Body is not wet; bindings (could indicate Homicide vs. Suicide); history of major depression or suicide attempts; found near a bridge or cliff

Applicable Scene Types

◆ *Intoxication / Overdose*
◆ *Suicide*

ENVIRONMENTAL INJURIES

ELECTROCUTION

Accident

Indicators

Electricians, maintenance men, and copper thieves have a higher chance of getting electrocuted. Physical evidence of an electrocution include burns and burn marks. Signs at the scene include: electrical equipment/tools near the body; signs of repair of electrical devices; damaged extension cords; or a ladder near an outdoor power source.

Key Questions

1. What is the suspected power source?
2. What is the current (amps) and voltage (volts) (if known)?
3. Is the ground wet or dry in the area of the suspected electrocution?

Scene Procedures

1. Request local fire department, power/utility company, or electrician to turn off the power and/or any electrical devices.
2. Photograph the suspected power source or electrical device.
3. Photograph any involved extension cords or any exposed wires.
4. Photograph any sources of ignition near the body.
5. Photograph any UL (Underwriters Laboratories) label or markings.
6. Collect the suspected device(s) (if portable) and involved electrical cords for further examination.
7. Examine the clothing and body for burns, especially the hands and feet.
8. Photograph burn defects on clothing, accessories and body.
9. Collect clothing items that fell off or were removed (gloves, hat, shoes).
10. Lock and seal the residence (if the incident occurred indoors).

Applicable Scene Types

◆ *Work-Related*

HYPERTHERMIA

Accident

Indicators

Hyperthermia should be considered in the summer months especially during environmental heat waves. Concern should be raised when the body is found outdoors; when utilities are shut off; when no alternative cooling sources are in use; when the decedent was exercising or laboring prior to collapse; and when the decedent had symptoms of heat stroke. Cocaine and certain antidepressants may induce hyperthermia.

Key Questions

1. What was the estimated or recorded temperature?

2. Was the indoor temperature uncomfortably warm when first responders entered?

3. Has the environment been changed by first responders to make it cooler?

4. Is the home cooling system working?

5. Are alternate cooling sources present?

    a. Are windows and doors open?

6. If decedent was laboring or exercising outdoors, for how long?

    a. Did decedent have specific complaints afterward?

7. Are there medications or illicit drugs on scene?

    a. Such as antidepressants or cocaine

Scene Procedures

1. Photograph the air conditioning unit and temperature reading (thermostat/thermometer).
2. Photograph alternate cooling sources.

HYPOTHERMIA

Accident

Indicators

Hypothermia should be considered when utilities are shut off; when found indoors with no heat source or outdoors during cooler weather with no trauma; when found nude outdoors (paradoxical undressing). Alcoholics are at higher risk of hypothermia.

Key Questions

1. What was the estimated or recorded temperature?
2. Was the indoor temperature uncomfortably cold when first responders entered?
3. Has the environment been changed by first responders to make it warmer?
4. Is the home heating system working?
5. Is the body frozen?
6. Are excessive wrappings, blankets, or extra layers of clothing in use?
7. Are the decedent's clothing wet?

Scene Procedures

Indoor

1. Photograph alternate heating sources/equipment.

Outdoor

1. If the body is nude, search for clothing in the immediate area.

2. If the decedent was missing for a few days, record the general weather conditions for that time frame.

FIRES

Accident, Suicide, Homicide

Indicators

When a body is discovered inside or near a burning structure, including an automobile, investigators may find thermal injuries including burns and charring. Prolonged exposure to fire will produce skin splitting, a pugilistic pose, consumption of tissue and bone beginning with the extremities, and artifactual fractures of bones. Inhalation of heavy smoke will produce the appearance of soot in and around the mouth and nasal passages.

Key Questions

1. How was the body found?
   a. Exact location and position?
   b. Close to a doorway or other exit?
   c. Was the body moved, removed or damaged during firefighting operations?
   d. Was anything on top of the body when it was found?

2. Is there a known or suspected ORIGIN of the fire? Where is it?

3. Is there a known or suspected CAUSE of the fire? What is it?

a. What physical evidence supports the preliminary *cause* (smoking materials, gas cans)?

b. Is there any evidence of an accelerant being used?

4. In general, what type of fire damage is present (smoke, burn, both)?

5. Any previous police or fire calls to this address? When and why?

6. Was anyone else present at the time of the fire?

7. Does the decedent smoke?

8. Any medical or cognitive conditions that would impede escape from the fire?

9. Were there smoke/fire alarms in the home? Location(s):

a. What was the operational status of the alarms?

Scene Procedures

1. Photograph items on the body.

2. Photograph sources of ignition near the body (smoking materials, space heaters, electrical).

3. Photograph fire/smoke alarms in relation to the decedent (if present).

4. Secure the hands in clean paper bags with rubber bands or tape in homicides, suspicious deaths or to preserve finger-prints when skin is de-gloving.

5. Discuss collection of clothing remnants with fire investigator/marshal.

📭 Red-Flags

Trauma inconsistent with thermal injury; firearms or shells/ casings near the body; blood pools near the body; found inside trunk of burned-out automobile

Applicable Scene Types

◆ *Suicide*

FIREARMS-RELATED DEATHS

Suicide, Homicide, Accident

Indicators

There will be a gunshot wound to the body. Possible firearms and casings/shells may be found on scene.

Key Questions

1. Handguns

    a. What type of firearm (if on scene)?

    b. Make/Model /Caliber/Serial number

    c. Who owns the firearm?

    d. What was the original location/position of the firearm?

    e. Has the firearm been moved and by whom?

    f. Are there other firearms on scene?

2. Shotguns

    a. What type of shotgun?

        i. Action type (pump, break, auto-loading).

        ii. Single or double barrel.

     b.   Was a shotgun cup/wadding found?

     c.   Was an object used to fire the shotgun?

3.   What type of ammunition (make and caliber/gauge)?

4.   How many unfired round(s)?

5.   How many fired rounds (spent casings)?

6.   Are there any other bullet defects in nearby objects?

7.   Were there any intervening objects (pillow, blanket, etc.)?

8.   Is there any firearm cleaning equipment on scene?

9.   Was the decedent right or left handed? (Suicide or Accident)

10.   Was the decedent familiar with firearms? (Suicide or Accident)

Scene Procedures

1.   Photograph the hands and feet (if applicable).

2.   Secure the hands and feet (if necessary) in clean paper bags with rubber bands or tape.

3.   Account for all fired rounds (test fires, intermediary objects, etc.).

4.   Photograph

     a.   Bullet defects in nearby objects.

     b.   The firearm (if present) in relationship to the body. NOTE: Ensure that the firearm is made safe/cleared by law enforcement personnel.

     c.   Fired casings in relationship to the body.

     d.   Ammunition near the body.

     e.   Cleaning equipment (when applicable).

     f.   Relevant bloodstain patterns.

     g.   One photo depicting items placed into the firearms evidence box (Suicides and Accidents).

5.   Evidence in a homicide investigation that's not on the body must be collected by law enforcement.

⚑ Red-Flags

Other types of trauma

Applicable Scene Types

◆   *Suicide*

IN-CUSTODY

Accident, Suicide, Homicide

Indicators

Any death while jailed, incarcerated or during law enforcement activity.

DURING LAW ENFORCEMENT ACTIVITY

Key Questions

1.   What was the reason the decedent was stopped, detained, or arrested?

2.   What are the details of the incident?

3.   Is there video footage of the incident?

4.   Were less lethal options used (pepper spray / electroshock device / bean bags)?

5.   Were restraints used?

Scene Procedures

1. Ask the officer or jailer to describe the encounter.
2. Request a copy of all available video footage.
3. Photograph of scale demonstrating relevant heights.
4. If hanging, photograph any ligature, anchor point, and point of suspension.

Applicable Scene Types

- *Blunt Force Injuries*
- *Firearms-Related*
- *Hanging*
- *In-Custody - Restraints*
- *Intoxication / Overdose*
- *Suicide*

JAIL OR PRISON

Key Questions

1. What was their date of booking or entry into prison/jail?
2. What were the charges?
3. Have they had any face-to-face visitation in the past 24 hours?
4. What was their cell arrangement (shared cell / holding / isolation / open dormitory)?
5. Has anything been removed from the scene or cell?
6. Was the decedent involved in a physical altercation?
7. Was he/she recently given prescription medication? What time?
8. Was he/she given any sedatives or other medications by medical staff?

9.   Any recent infirmary/medical visits?

10. Is there video footage?

Scene Procedures

1.   Ask the officer or jailer to describe the encounter.

2.   Request a copy of all available video footage.

3.   Request a copy of pertinent log-book entries (suicide watch, medication administration, etc.).

Applicable Scene Types

◆   *Blunt Force Injuries*
◆   *Hanging*
◆   *In-Custody - Restraints*
◆   *Intoxication / Overdose*
◆   *Suicide*

RESTRAINTS

Homicide

Indicators

The decedent was restrained by police officers during arrest or by correctional officers while imprisoned.

Key Questions

1.   How many persons were involved in the restraint process?

2.   What type of restraints or choke holds were used?

    a.   Was the decedent's nose or mouth obstructed or neck compressed during restraint?

3.   In what position(s) was he/she restrained?

4.   Where was he/she restrained (specific location) and for how long?

5.   Did he/she demonstrate signs of consciousness after restraint?

Scene Procedures

1.   Ask the officer or jailer to describe the encounter.

2.   Photograph restraints.

3.   Request a copy of all available video footage.

INTOXICATION / OVERDOSE

ALCOHOL ABUSE

Natural, Accident

Indicators

Anytime there's excessive alcohol at the scene, investigators should consider acute alcohol intoxication as the cause of death. It's important to differentiate acute versus chronic alcohol abuse. Acute alcohol poisoning incidents present following an all-night party or binge drinking with friends. Chronic abusers tend to have a thin, disheveled appearance and may be jaundiced secondary to liver cirrhosis. Alcoholics frequently fall and it's typical to observe a number of contusions on the body in various stages of healing. The scene may present as suspicious or violent due to a large amount of hemorrhage from ruptured esophageal varices. Overturned or broken furniture is sometimes encountered because the decedent fell while intoxicated.

Key Questions

1. What type, how much, and where was the alcohol found at the scene?

2. When no alcohol is found, are they sober or were they drinking at another location?

3. What is their beverage of choice, how much, and how often do they drink?

4. How long have they been abusing?

5. Has the decedent ever received treatment or been institutionalized?

    a. Where, how long, and when were they released?

    b. If they were recently released, did he or she exhibit symptoms of withdrawal?

6. How long have they been sober?

    a. Recent life events that may have triggered relapse?

Scene Procedures

1. Photograph evidence of alcohol consumption.

2. Describe beverages near the body.

📕 Red-Flags

Position of the body, illicit drugs, prescription drugs.

Applicable Scene Types

◆ *Asphyxia - Positional*
◆ *Blunt Force Injuries*
◆ *Hypothermia*
◆ *Falls from Standing*

- *Falls Down Stairs*
- *Falls or Jump from Height*

ILLICIT DRUGS

Natural, Accident, Suicide (rare)

Indicators

Physical findings include track marks, acute punctures, and foam cones. Remnants of illicit drugs and paraphernalia are often found on or near the body and in the trash.

Key Questions

1. What type of illicit drugs were found and where?

2. What paraphernalia, if any, was present?

3. What drugs is the decedent known to abuse?

   a. How do they use / administer the substance? (smoke, snort, inject, swallow)

4. How long have they been abusing?

   a. Was there a life event that triggered the drug abuse?

5. Has the decedent ever received treatment or been institutionalized for drug abuse?

   a. Where, how long admitted, and when were they released?

   b. If recently released, did he or she exhibit symptoms of withdrawal?

6. If sober, for how long?

   a. Any recent life events that may have triggered relapse?

7. Has the decedent had prior overdoses?

    a. When, what substance, and where treated?

8. Any indication that this is an intentional overdose?

Scene Procedures

1. Photograph all suspected illicit drugs and paraphernalia.

2. Describe drugs and paraphernalia near the body.

3. Photograph foam cone if it's not clearly shown in the mug-shot photo.

4. Collect drugs and paraphernalia in separate bags or containers and place all items collectively into a larger bag or container for transport.

    a. Place all items inside the body bag and seal the body bag.

    b. Complete an illicit drugs and paraphernalia inventory form.

    c. Follow agency protocols for submission of drugs and paraphernalia for testing or storage.

Red-Flags

Suicide note, prior suicide attempts, empty prescription bottles near the body, and psychiatric conditions. When another person injected the decedent the case should be investigated as a homicide.

Applicable Scene Types

◆ *Alcohol Abuse*
◆ *Suicide*

INHALANT / VOLATILE SUBSTANCE ABUSE

Accident, Suicide

Indicators

Chemical sprays or liquids found outside normal storage areas. Empty chemical containers may be found under the bed, in the trash or in another hiding spot. Physical findings may include: foam cones, frost bite on the face, or paint on the face or clothing. Family members or friends may deny that the decedent huffs or abuses inhalants, but they may disclose that the decedent frequently coughs, sneezes, is drowsy, hallucinates, has nosebleeds, or has seizures.

Key Questions

1. Was a potential inhalant / volatile substance found near the body?

    a. What is it? What form is it in?

2. Does the decedent have a history of inhalant / volatile substance abuse?

    a. What method do they use (huffing, sniffing, spraying, bagging, hooding)?

    b. Hooding is placing a bag over the head and spraying or huffing the chemical.

Scene Procedures

1. Photograph suspected inhalants/volatiles including the brand name.

2. Photograph the nozzle, fabric, and/or bag used to inhale vapors.

3. Record the name of the manufacturer.

4. Inspect trash cans, closets, and underneath beds for empty containers.

5. Search for receipts for the purchase of chemicals.

6. Collect the suspected inhalant and follow agency protocols for submission.

🚩 Red-Flags

Plastic bag over the head could be "Final Exit" or homicide.

Applicable Scene Types

◆ *Asphyxia - Plastic Bag ("Final Exit")*
◆ *Suicide*

PRESCRIPTION DRUGS

Accident, Suicide

Indicators

Pain relievers, central nervous system depressants, and stimulants are commonly abused and should raise the question of a possible overdose. Discord in the pill inventory and/or a history of prior overdoses support the conclusion of an overdose. Possession of another person's medication or unlabeled prescription bottles may also indicate abuse. A foam cone is often present in an opiate overdose.

Key Questions

1. Are commonly abused prescriptions at the scene (list on pg. 78)?

2. Are prescriptions present which are not in the decedent's name?

3. Is there evidence the decedent obtained controlled substances from multiple health care practitioners ("doctor shopping")?

4. Are the medications self-administered or administered by others?

   a. Are the medications secured? Explain.

5. Does the decedent have a history of prescription overdose?

   a. When, what prescription(s), and where was he or she treated?

6. Any indication this is an intentional overdose?

Scene Procedures

1. Photograph prescription bottles at the scene especially those near the body.

2. Collect prescription medications in accordance with agency policies.

3. Record the following into the Medicine Inventory/Chain of Custody form:

   (1) Drug name

   (2) Date filled

   (3) Quantity prescribed

   (4) Number of pills remaining

   (5) Dosage directions

   (6) Full name of prescribing physician

4. Do not collect medications not in the decedent's name.

   a. Note the drug name and record in the report.

5. Collect unlabeled prescription bottles containing pills.

🏴 Red-Flags

Suicide note or prior suicide attempts.

Applicable Scene Types

◆ *Suicide*

MOTOR VEHICLE ACCIDENTS

Accident, Suicide (rare)

Indicators

The decedent is found inside a vehicle or on the roadway / road-side at the scene of a crash. Physical findings may include: blunt force injuries, dicing injuries from broken auto glass, and seat belt pattern abrasions. Never presume a collision was an accident particularly when the decedent's vehicle was the only automobile involved.

Key Questions

1. What are the details of the accident?
   a. What were the weather, road and lighting conditions?
   b. What type of roadway (concrete / asphalt / gravel)? Describe.
   c. Were the brakes applied prior to impact?
      i. Length of skid-marks?
   d. What was the estimated speed and/or posted speed limit?
   e. Were there traffic control lights or noteworthy signage in the immediate area?

    f. Did the vehicle rollover?

    g. If the body is outside the vehicle, was he/she ejected or removed by someone?

    h. Was there evidence of alcohol or drug use or distracted driving?

2. What was the decedent's position within his/her vehicle?

    (Driver / Passenger/ Backseat)

    a. Was he/she wearing a seatbelt?

        i. If yes, what was the condition of the seatbelt?

    b. Was the vehicle equipped with airbags? Did they deploy?

    c. Who is the decedent's vehicle registered to?

3. What are the makes, models, and styles of vehicles involved?

    a. Where was the major damage on each vehicle?

    b. How many occupants were inside the vehicle(s)?

4. Are all involved vehicles still at the scene?

    a. If not, is this a hit-and-run?

Scene Procedures

1. Photograph all four sides of the vehicle.

    a. Capture the license plate in at least one photo.

2. Photograph opposing views of the vehicle's interior depicting the deceased.

3. Photograph closest intersection or landmark in relation to the accident.

4. Photograph relevant skid marks, point of impact, and damage on the roadway.

5. Photograph the seatbelt, airbags, or other restraints (if relevant).

6. Use extreme caution regarding identification when multiple occupants are involved.

    a. If others were injured, obtain their condition and hospital information.

🚩 Red-Flags

Single vehicle versus a fixed object could be a suicide.

Applicable Scene Types

◆ *Fires*
◆ *Seizures*
◆ *Suicide*

AUTO VS. PEDESTRIAN

Accident, Suicide, Homicide

Indicators

The decedent was found on the road or near the roadway with blunt force injuries. The location of injuries provide clues as to the decedent's position when struck and occasionally clues to the general class or type of offending automobile. Footwear is often dislodged and thrown a great distance if the decedent was standing when struck. Physical findings may include: bumper injuries, road rash abrasions, pattern injuries, traumatic amputations, and pattern markings/impressions on the clothing.

Key Questions

1. Was the incident witnessed?

2.   What was the decedent's position on the roadway when struck (if known)?

3.   Did the vehicle flee the scene?

4.   Refer to Key Questions for Motor Vehicle Accidents.

Scene Procedures

1.   Measure the bumper height when striking vehicle is present.

2.   Follow MVA Scene Procedures

🚩 Red-Flags

Decedent was lying on the roadway. Decedent was suicidal.

Applicable Scene Types

◆   *Motor Vehicle Accidents*
◆   *Suicide*

SEIZURES

Natural, Accident, Homicide

Indicators

Death due to seizures is a diagnosis of exclusion. The primary medicolegal concern is when seizures are the result of head trauma or drug-induced hypoxia. When there's a documented history of seizures, investigators should look for seizure medication, white or blood tinged foam, disrupted bedding, tongue biting, and discharge of urine or feces.

Key Questions

1. What is the underlying cause?

2. Are the seizures generally controlled by medication?

3. Is the decedent compliant with taking medications?

4. What was the date of or the decedent's age at first seizure?

5. What type of seizures (grand mal, absence, myoclonic, clonic, tonic, atonic, ideopathic)?

   a. Are the seizures the result of alcohol or drug withdrawal?

   b. If type is unknown, ask about the decedent's symptoms before, during and after a seizure spell?

6. How frequently does he or she have seizures?

7. How long do the seizures typically last?

8. Has there been a recent change in seizure activity? Describe.

Scene Procedures

1. Obtain the seizure history from the most knowledgeable witness(es).

2. Note pill discrepancies for seizure medications.

⚑ Red-Flags

Seizure-like activity could be the result of recent or remote head trauma which could be a delayed homicide.

Applicable Scene Types

◆ *Asphyxia - Positional*
◆ *Alcohol Abuse*
◆ *Blunt Force Injuries*

- *Drowning*
- *Falls Down Stairs*
- *Falls from Standing*
- *Falls or Jump from Height*
- *Fires*
- *Intoxication / Overdose*
- *Motor Vehicle Accidents*
- *Sudden Unexpected Infant Death Investigations (SUIDI)*

SHARP FORCE INJURIES

Accident, Suicide, or Homicide

Indicators

Physical findings of this type of death include incised and stab wounds. Cutting injuries have clean margins with no tissue bridging or abrasions. Defense injuries may be on the hands, arms and occasionally the legs. Hesitation marks should raise the possibility that the injuries were self-inflicted.

Key Questions

1. Was a suspected sharp instrument found?
    a. What is it and where was it found?
    b. Was it moved? By whom?
    c. Is there apparent blood on it?
    d. If the instrument is a knife, what type (single or double-edge, serrated, other-explain)?
    e. Were any similar sharp instruments found?
2. Are there any apparent defense injuries or hesitation marks?
3. SUICIDE: Was the decedent right or left handed?

Scene Procedures

1. When present, photograph, obtain measurements, and collect the sharp instrument in accordance with agency protocol.

2. Photograph the knife or cutting instrument prior to collection as well as in the knife box after collection.

3. Photograph any similar sharp instruments present at the scene (knife block, utensil drawer).

4. Never remove a sharp instrument that's embedded in the body.

   a. Cover the handle with a paper bag.

5. Photograph apparent defense injuries or hesitation marks.

6. Secure the hands in clean paper bags with rubber bands or tape.

Applicable Scene Types

◆ *Suicide*

SUDDEN UNEXPECTED INFANT DEATH INVESTIGATIONS (SUIDI)

Natural, Accident, Homicide, Undetermined

Indicators

Previously healthy infant (12 months or less) pronounced at home or in the emergency room.

Key Questions

1. Is there evidence of asphyxia (overlay, wedging, and nose/mouth obstruction)?

2. Was the sleep surface being shared with another person or animal?

3. Were there unsafe sleeping conditions (ex. couch, adult bed, pillows, etc.)?

4. How was the infant *placed*?

    a. Was the airway potentially obstructed?

5. How was the infant *found*?

    a. Was the airway potentially obstructed?

6. Recent fall or other injury?

7. History of acute life-threatening events (apnea, seizures, difficulty breathing)?

8. Prior sibling deaths?

    a. What was the cause?

9. Recent changes to the infant's diet (ex. introduction of solid foods)?

10. Religious, cultural or ethnic remedies?

11. Has a previous report been made to Child Protective Services or police?

<u>Scene Procedures</u>

1. Refer to the CDC's guidelines.

2. Conduct investigation in collaboration with law enforcement.

3. Photograph the infant at the hospital.

4. Conduct interviews with involved parties.

5. Conduct doll re-enactment at the residence.

    a. Photograph placed and found positions with special attention to the airway.

6. Photograph the sleep surface in layers.

7. Photograph other potential sleep environments (crib, adult bed, car seat, swing).

8. Photograph any stains on bedding or caregivers clothing.

9. Follow agency protocols for collecting items from the scene.

    a. Request police collect formula bottle(s) and medications including over the counter.

10. Document any parent/caregiver prescriptions.

11. Report case to Child Protective Services.

    a. Record reference number, history, type of allegations, and findings/outcomes.

Red-Flags

History of prior infant deaths in the family; child in the care of someone with no biological relationship (i.e. mother's boyfriend); caregiver with mental health or substance abuse problems; history of prior trauma to the infant; obvious trauma; open cases with CPS; no prenatal care

Applicable Scene Types

- *Abuse or Neglect of a Child or Adolescent*
- *Asphyxia - Compression (Traumatic)*
- *Asphyxia - Positional*
- *Drowning*
- *Hyperthermia*
- *Hypothermia*

WORK-RELATED

Accident

Indicators

The decedent became unresponsive or was injured while at work; including individuals who are self-employed. Natural deaths occur frequently while working, but trauma and occupational exposure must be ruled-out.

Key Questions

1. What was the decedent's assignment at the time of the incident?

    a. If witnessed, what happened?

    b. What was the decedent's experience or training level at this job assignment?

2. What is his or her work schedule?

3. What is the decedent's job title?

4. What are the job duties?

5. What time did he/she report to work on the date of the incident?

6. What is the name of company (employer), address, and phone number?

7. Is there surveillance video of the incident?

    a. Who is the point of contact to obtain the video?

8. How long has the decedent worked for the company?

    a. How long in his or her current position?

9. Has anyone else been sickened (now or previously)?

10.   Has OSHA or appropriate state agency been notified?

Scene Procedures

1.   Photograph personal safety equipment, connections, and/or OSHA required equipment.

2.   Photograph safety signage and/or labeling.

3.   Photograph electrical devices or cords near the decedent.

4.   Photograph equipment/machinery the decedent was operating.

5.   Collect clothing that fell off or was removed from the body (i.e. gloves, hard hats).

6.   Disconnect lanyards or other connections at the body (leave lanyards connected to equipment).

Applicable Scene Types

◆   *Asphyxia*
◆   *Blunt Force Injuries*
◆   *Carbon Monoxide (CO)*
◆   *Falls Down Stairs*
◆   *Falls from Standing*
◆   *Falls or Jump from Height*
◆   *Fires*
◆   *Electrocution*
◆   *Sharp Force Injuries*

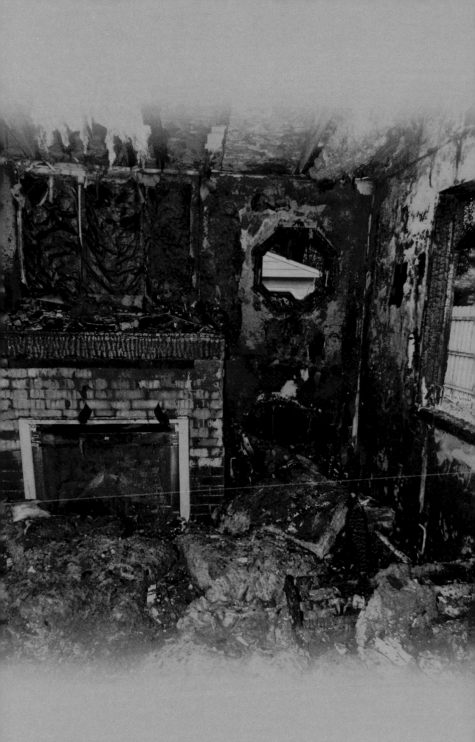

APPENDIX

COMMONLY ABUSED PRESCRIPTION DRUGS

Generic Name (Brand name)	Treats	Class
Amphetamine (Dexadrine®, Adderall®)	ADHD	Stimulant
Alprazolam (Xanax®)	Psych disorders	Benzodiazepine
Amitriptyline (Elavil®)	Psych disorders, pain	Tricyclic antidepressant
Carisoprodol (Soma®)	Pain and stiffness	Muscle relaxant
Citalopram (Celexa®)	Psych disorders	SSRI
Clonazepam (Klonopin®)	Psych disorders, seizures	Benzodiazepine
Codeine - liquid	Pain, cough	Opioid
Cyclobenzaprine (Flexeril®)	Pain and stiffness	Muscle relaxant
Diazepam (Valium®)	Psych disorders, seizures	Benzodiazepine
Doxepin (Sinequan®)	Psych disorders	Tricyclic antidepressant
Eszopiclone (Lunesta®)	Sleep disorder	Hypnotic
Fentanyl (Duragesic®, Actiq®)	Pain	Opioid
Fluoxetine (Prozac®)	Psych disorders	SSRI
Hydrocodone (Vicodin®)	Pain	Opioid
Hydromorphone (Dilaudid®)	Pain	Opioid
Lorazepam (Ativan®)	Psych disorders	Benzodiazepine
Methadone – liquid	Pain, Opiate addiction	Analgesic, Opioid
Methocarbamol (Robaxin®)	Pain	Muscle relaxant
Methylphenidate (Concerta®, Ritalin®)	ADHD	Stimulant
Oxycodone (oxycontin®)	Pain	Opioid
Oxymorphone (Opana®)	Pain	Opioid
Percocet (acetaminophen + Oxycodone)	Pain	Opioid
Phenobarbital Nembutal®)	Anxiety, Seizures	Barbiturates
Propoxyphene (Darvon®)	Pain	Opioid
Sertraline (Zoloft®)	Psych disorders	SSRI
Temazepam (Restoril®)	Psych disorders	Benzodiazepine
Tramadol (Ultram®)	Pain and stiffness	Muscle relaxant
Trazodone (Oleptro®)	Psych and sleep disorders	Serotonin antagonist
Triazolam (Halcion®)	Insomnia	Benzodiazepine
Zaleplon (Sonata®)	Sleep disorder	Hypnotic
Zolpidem (Ambien®)	Sleep disorder	Benzodiazepine

GLOSSARY

Abrasion: a wound caused by superficial damage to the skin, no deeper than the epidermis

Accident: due to injury when there is no evidence of intent to harm

Anterior: in front of

Atrophy: wasting away

Battle's Sign: is bruising behind the ear, an indication of fracture of middle cranial fossa of the skull, and may suggest underlying brain trauma

Blanching: to press blood away and wait for return, such as blanching of lividity and return of blood

Cause of Death: refers to the disease or injury that initiated the train of events leading directly to death or the circumstances

Circumstance of Death: a fact or condition connected with or relevant to an event or action leading to death

Congenital: a condition that is present at birth

Contusion: is a type of hematoma of tissue in which capillaries and sometimes venules are damaged by trauma, allowing blood to seep, hemorrhage, into the surrounding tissues

Decomposition: is the process by which organic substances are broken down into simpler forms of matter

Dicing: multiple cubed lacerations of the skin seen in MVA victims who strike shattered tempered glass

Distal: away from the point of insertion

Ecchymoses: hemorrhages beneath the skin (larger than petechiae)

Emaciated: generalized wasting away

Exsanguination: marked internal or external loss of blood

Foam Cone: a foam like substance coming from either the nose, mouth or both

Fouling (Soot): residue of completely burned powder, dust-like (wipes off)

Furrow / Ligature Mark: a groove in the tissue created by the ligature which is pale in color, but later becomes yellowish or yellow/brown and hard like parchment due to the drying of the slightly abraded skin.

Hematoma: a mass (collection) of blood

Hemoptysis: spitting up blood or blood-tinged sputum from the respiratory tract. It occurs when tiny blood vessels that line the lung airways are broken

Hesitation Wounds: superficial, sharp, forced straight-line marks or scars at the elbows, neck/throat, and wrists found on the body of victims, typical of suicidal injuries

Homicide: due to a volitional act of another person with the intent to cause fear, harm or death

Incised Wound: a wound characterized by a clean cut, as by a sharp instrument

Inferior: below

Laceration: is a wound that is produced by the tearing of soft body tissue. This type of wound is often irregular and jagged (tissue bridging)

Livor Mortis: is the settling of the blood in the lower (dependent) portion of the body, causing a purplish red discoloration of the skin

Manner of Death: is how the death came about; a judgment based on circumstances surrounding the event

Medial: the middle

Natural: due entirely to natural disease processes

Paradoxical Undressing: is a phenomenon sometimes seen in persons dying from hypothermia in which the decedent removes all or part of their clothing secondary to a *sensation* of overheating.

Petechia; plural **petechiae:** is a pinpoint red or purple spot on the skin, caused by a minor hemorrhage

Posterior: behind or back

Prone: lying face down

Proximal: toward the point of insertion or the main part of the body

Purge Fluid: is the decayed reddish - brown foul smelling fluid leaving the body (Sometimes fluid is confused for blood)

Putrefaction: is the decomposition of proteins in a process that results in the eventual breakdown of cohesion between tissues and the liquefaction of most organs. It is caused due to bacterial or fungal decomposition of organic matter and results in production of obnoxious odors

Raccoon Eyes: a description for bilateral periorbital accumulations of blood often associated with fractures of the skull

Rigor Mortis: is one of the recognizable signs of death, caused by chemical changes in the muscles after death, causing the limbs of the body to become stiff and difficult to move or manipulate. In humans, it commences after about three to four hours, reaches maximum stiffness after 12 hours, and gradually dissipates from approximately 24 hours after death

Stippling (Tattooing): unburned powder and debris, causing punctate abrasions on target: larger and heavier so travels farther (Does not wipe off)

Subcutaneous Marbling: the outlines of the blood vessels under the skin seen in decomposed bodies

Suicide: due to injury that occurred with the intent to induce self-harm or cause one's own death

Superior: above

Supine: lying on the back with face upward

Tache Noir: is one of the ocular signs of death in which a reddish brown discoloration is transversely arranged across the sclera. It occurs when the eyes are not completely closed so that the sclera is exposed to air

Tardieu Spots: small hemorrhages from ruptured blood vessels on the extremities that occur after the body has been in a dependent position

Track Mark: a series of dark scars that follow the veins in individuals who chronically inject drugs

Undetermined: inadequate information regarding the circumstances of death to determine manner

Washerwoman Skin: wrinkled skin of the hands and feet seen in bodies recovered from water

IMPORTANT PHONE NUMBERS

Agency: _Cuyahoga County Medical Examiner 's Office_

Address: _11001 Cedar Ave ., Cleveland , Ohio 44106_

Phone _(216) 721-5610_

Agency:_____

Address:_____

Phone:_____

Agency:_____

Address:_____

Phone:_____

Agency:_____

Address:_____

Phone:_____

Agency:_____

Address:_____

Phone:_____

Agency:_____

Address:_____

Phone:_____

Agency:_____

Address:_____

Phone:_____

Agency:_____

Address:_____

Phone:_____

Agency:_____

Address:_____

Phone:_____

Agency:_____

Address:_____

Phone:_____

Agency:_____

Address:_____

Phone:_____

Agency:_____

Address:_____

Phone:_____

The Cuyahoga County Medical Examiner's Office *Medicolegal Death Investigation Field Guide'* has been completed with contributions from the following:

Thomas P. Gilson, M.D. .... Medical Examiner

Joseph P. Stopak, D-ABMDI .... Manager of Investigation and Morgue Operations

Michelle Fox, D-ABMDI .... Medicolegal Death Investigator II

Christopher Harris .... Communications Specialist

Jan Mannion.. Medical Secretaries Supervisor

Mike Schaedler, D-ABMDI .... Medicolegal Death Investigator II

Kate M. Snyder, CFPH........................... Chief Forensic Photographer

Amanda Wallace, D-ABMDI .... Medicolegal Death Investigator/PA

Justin Wilson, D-ABMDI .... Medicolegal Death Investigator

Erin Worrell, D-ABMDI........................... Medicolegal Death Investigator II

Previous Version Contributors:

Dan Morgan, F-ABMDI......................... Chief Investigator (Former)

James Wentzel .... Chief Forensic Photographer (Retired)

Cindie Carroll-Pankhurst, D-ABMDI............Medicolegal Death Investigator (Retired)